AYESHA MUJAWAR

Hope in the darkness

Overcoming depression

Contents

One

Major reasons causing depression

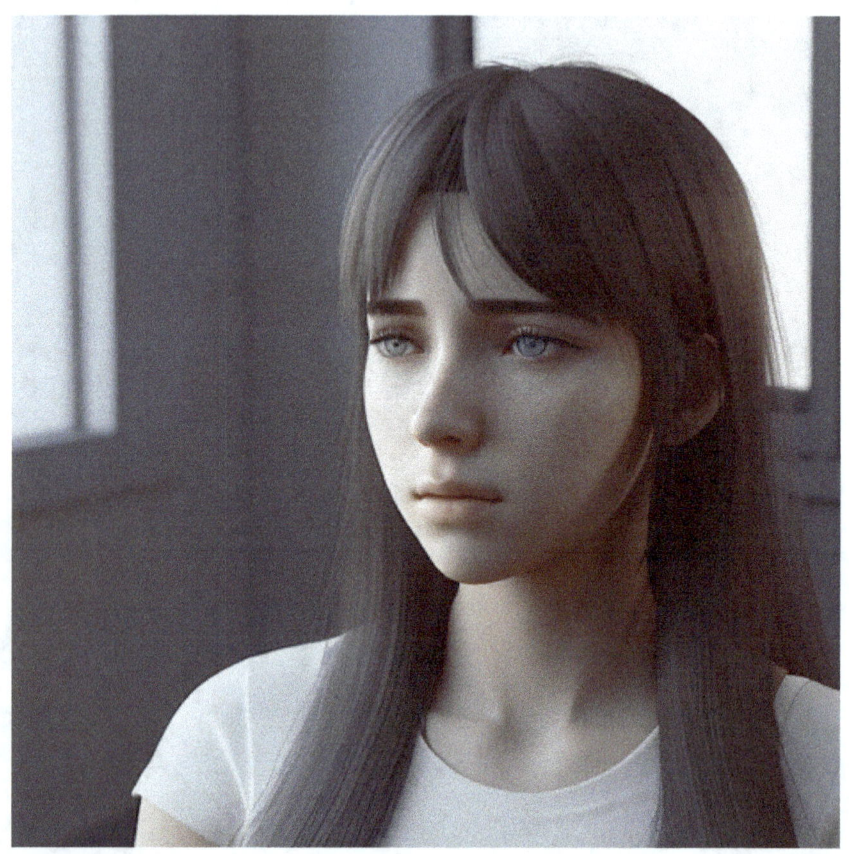

Reasons causing depression in teenager :

Depression is a serious mental health issue that can affect people of all ages, including teenagers. Adolescence is a time of significant changes and challenges, and it can be a difficult time for many teenagers. There are several reasons why depression occurs in teenagers. In this essay, we will discuss some of the major reasons that cause depression in teenagers.

1. Social Media: Nowadays, social media plays a big role in the lives of

teenagers. Social media can be a great way to connect with others, but it can also lead to feelings of isolation and low self-esteem. Comparing oneself with others on social media can lead to negative self-esteem and the feeling of not being good enough, which can trigger depression.

2. Academic Pressure: Pressure to perform well academically is a common cause of depression in teenagers. The pressure to do well can be overwhelming, leading to stress and feelings of inadequacy, which are triggered by the high expectations of parents, teachers, and society.

3. Family Problems: Many teenagers experience turbulence in their family relationships, which can lead to depression. Some family issues that can cause depression may include divorce, separation, or emotional abuse. Teenagers who experience these issues may feel isolated and alone, leading to depression.

4. Trauma: Traumatic events such as the loss of a loved one or experiencing a serious illness can lead to depression in teenagers. If left unaddressed, these traumatic events can lead to long-term negative effects on mental health.

5. Hormonal Changes: Hormonal changes during puberty can also affect mental health. During adolescence, many teenagers experience hormonal changes that can lead to mood swings and emotional instability, which are often associated with depression.

6. Substance Abuse: Many teenagers may experiment with drugs or alcohol to cope with depression or other mental health issues. However, it can become a vicious cycle where substance abuse can adversely effect their mental health.

Causes of depression in adults:

some of the major reasons that can cause depression in adults.

1. Genetic Factors: Research has shown that depression can run in families, indicating a genetic component to the condition. Having a family history of depression can increase one's risk of developing the condition.

2. Life Events: Major life stressors such as the loss of a loved one, divorce, financial problems, or job loss can trigger depression in adults. These life events can cause significant emotional pain and lead to feelings of hopelessness and despair.

3. Chronic Illness: Adults living with chronic illnesses such as cancer, heart disease, or diabetes often experience depression as a result of the physical and emotional toll the conditions can take on their lives. Dealing with the consequences of a chronic illness can be overwhelming, leading to depression.

4. Substance Abuse: Adults who struggle with substance abuse, including alcohol and drugs, are at increased risk of developing depression. Substance abuse can disrupt brain chemistry and cause significant emotional distress, leading to depression.

5. Hormonal Changes: Women may experience depression as a result of hormone changes during menopause or after giving birth. These life transitions can cause fluctuations in hormone levels, leading to mood swings and depression.

6. Social Isolation: Adults who lack social connections or feel isolated

from others are at increased risk of developing depression. Living in isolation can lead to feelings of loneliness and hopelessness, leading to depression.

Reasons causing depression in elderly people:

1. Social Isolation: Elderly individuals who lack social connections or feel isolated from others are at increased risk of developing depression.

2. Chronic Health Conditions: Elderly individuals who have chronic health conditions, such as arthritis, diabetes, or heart disease, are at increased risk of developing depression.

3. Cognitive Decline: Elderly individuals who experience cognitive decline, such as Alzheimer's disease or dementia, are at increased risk of developing depression.

4. Loss of Independence: Elderly individuals who experience a loss of independence, such as mobility or the ability to complete daily tasks on their own, may experience depression.

5. Financial Strain: Elderly individuals who experience financial strain, such as retirement savings etc.

Here are some of the common stages of depression:

1. Mild depression: This is the earliest stage of depression, and it is characterized by feelings of sadness, low mood, and a lack of motivation. People in this stage may still be able to function in their daily lives, but they may find it more difficult to enjoy the things they used to.

2. Moderate depression: In this stage, the symptoms of depression become more severe. People may experience feelings of hopelessness and helplessness, and may have trouble concentrating or making decisions. They may also experience changes in appetite, sleep patterns, and energy levels.

3. Severe depression: Severe depression is the most intense stage of depression, and it can be debilitating. People in this stage may experience suicidal thoughts or behaviors, and may have difficulty functioning in their daily lives. They may also experience physical symptoms, such as headaches, stomachaches, and other aches and pains.

4. Recovery: With the right treatment and support, people with depression can recover and return to their normal lives. This stage is characterized by a reduction in symptoms, an improvement in mood and energy levels, and a return to normal functioning.

Conclusion

In conclusion, depression is a complex disorder that affects people across all age groups. It has no single cause but is usually a result of various factors that interact with mental health.

If depression is not recovered, it can have a significant impact on a person's life. Here are some of the potential consequences of untreated depression:

1. Impaired functioning: Depression can make it difficult for people to function in their daily lives. They may struggle with work or school, have trouble maintaining relationships, and find it hard to take care of themselves.

2. Physical health problems: Depression has been linked to a variety of physical health problems, including heart disease, diabetes, and chronic pain. People with depression may also be more susceptible to infections and illnesses.

3. Substance abuse: Depression can increase the risk of substance abuse and addiction. People with depression may turn to drugs or alcohol as a way of coping with their symptoms.

4. Relationship problems: Depression can strain relationships with family and friends. People with depression may withdraw from social activities and have difficulty communicating with others.

5. Suicidal thoughts or behaviors: Depression is a leading cause of suicide. People with depression may experience thoughts of self-harm or suicide, and may be at risk of attempting suicide if they do not receive treatment.

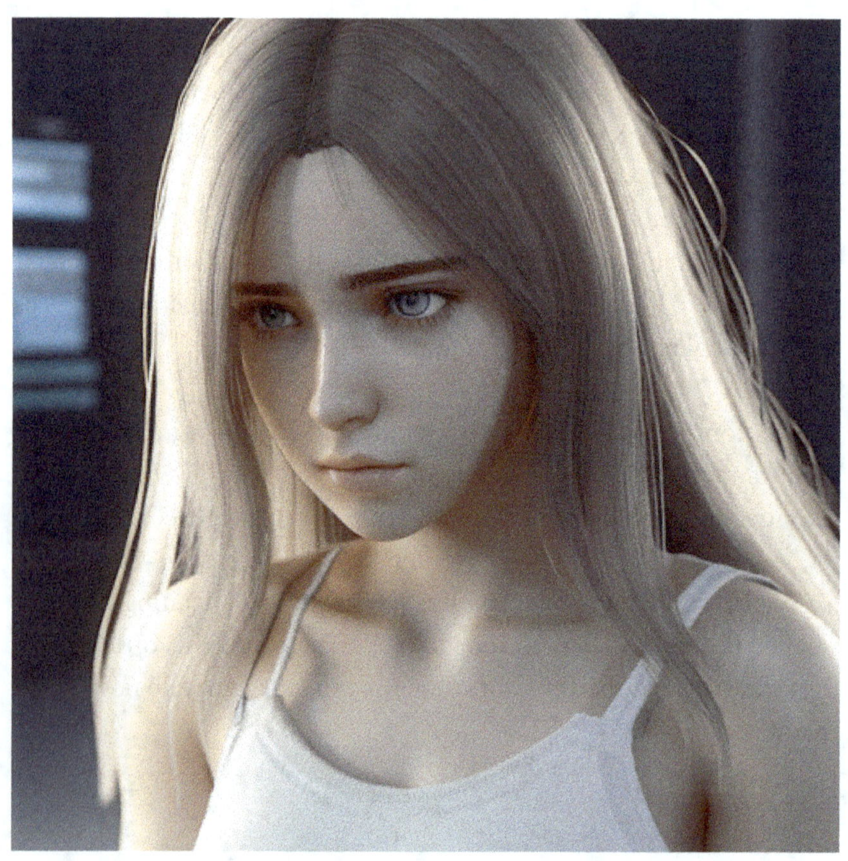

Two

Overcoming suicidal tendency

S uicidal tendency, also known as suicidal ideation, refers to the thoughts and feelings of wanting to end one's life. It is a serious mental health concern that can affect people of all ages, genders, and backgrounds. Suicidal thoughts can be triggered by a variety of factors, including depression, anxiety, trauma, and substance abuse. People who experience suicidal thoughts may feel hopeless, helpless, and overwhelmed, and may believe that there is no other way to escape their pain. It is important to recognize the signs of suicidal ideation and to seek help if you or someone you know is experiencing these thoughts. With the right support and treatment, it is possible to overcome suicidal tendencies and find hope and healing.Suicidal tendency is a complex and multifaceted issue, and it requires a compassionate and comprehensive approach to address it. It is important to understand that suicidal thoughts are not a sign of weakness or a character flaw. Rather, they are a symptom of a deeper mental health issue that needs to be addressed. It is also important to note that suicide is preventable, and that there are many resources available for people who are struggling with suicidal thoughts.

If you or someone you know is experiencing suicidal thoughts, it is important to seek help immediately. This may include reaching out to a mental health professional, contacting a crisis hotline, or seeking emergency medical care. It is also important to take steps to reduce access to lethal means, such as firearms or medications.

It is important to remember that suicidal thoughts are treatable, and that recovery is possible. With the right support and treatment, people who experience suicidal thoughts can learn to manage their symptoms and find hope and healing. It is never too late to seek help, and reaching out for support is a sign of strength and courage.

There are many effective treatments available for suicidal tendency, including therapy, medication, and support groups. Cognitive-behavioral therapy (CBT) is a common form of therapy that helps people identify and change negative thought patterns that contribute to suicidal thoughts. Medications such as antidepressants and mood stabilizers may also be used to help manage symptoms of depression and other mental health conditions that can contribute to suicidal thoughts.

In addition to professional treatment, there are many self-care strategies that can help reduce the risk of suicide. These may include getting regular exercise, eating a healthy diet, getting enough sleep, and practicing stress-reducing techniques such as meditation or yoga. It is also important to reach out to friends and family for support, and to seek out community resources such as support groups or social services.

If you are concerned about a loved one who may be experiencing suicidal thoughts, it is important to take their concerns seriously and to encourage them to seek help. You can offer to help them find a mental health professional, accompany them to appointments, or simply listen and offer support. Remember that suicidal thoughts are a medical emergency, and it is important to take action to keep your loved one safe.

In conclusion, suicidal tendency is a serious mental health issue that requires compassionate and comprehensive treatment. With the right support and treatment, people who experience suicidal thoughts can learn to manage their symptoms and find hope and healing. If you or someone you know is experiencing suicidal thoughts, it is important to seek help immediately. Remember that help is available, and that recovery is possible.

If suicidal tendency increases, it can have devastating consequences for individuals, families, and communities. Here are some of the potential consequences of an increase in suicidal tendency:

1. Higher suicide rates: An increase in suicidal tendency can lead to a higher number of suicides. Suicide is a leading cause of death worldwide, and an increase in suicidal thoughts and behaviors can lead to a corresponding increase in suicide rates.

2. Mental health crisis: An increase in suicidal tendency can also lead to a mental health crisis. Mental health professionals may be overwhelmed by the demand for services, and resources such as crisis hotlines and emergency mental health services may become overwhelmed.

3. Economic impact: Suicide can have a significant economic impact on families and communities. The loss of a loved one to suicide can

lead to lost income, medical expenses, and other financial burdens.

4. Social impact: Suicide can also have a significant social impact on families and communities. It can lead to feelings of guilt, shame, and stigma, and can strain relationships between family members and friends.

5. Long-term consequences: The effects of an increase in suicidal tendency can be long-lasting. Families and communities may struggle with the aftermath of suicide for years or even decades, and the trauma of suicide can be passed down from generation to generation.

It is important to recognize that suicidal tendency is a serious mental health issue that requires attention and action. It is important to take steps to reduce the risk of suicide, including seeking help for mental health issues, reducing access to lethal means, and promoting mental health awareness and education. With the right support and treatment, it is possible to prevent suicide and reduce the impact of suicidal tendency on individuals, families, and communities.

Overcoming suicidal tendencies while facing depression can be a difficult and complex process, but there are several strategies that can help. Here are some ways to overcome suicidal tendencies while facing depression:

1. Seek professional help: One of the most important steps in overcoming suicidal tendencies while facing depression is to seek professional help. A mental health professional can provide a diagnosis, develop a treatment plan, and offer support and guidance throughout the recovery process.

2. Take medication: In many cases, medication can be an effective treatment for depression and suicidal tendencies. Antidepressants and other medications can help regulate mood, reduce anxiety, and improve overall mental health.

3. Participate in therapy: Therapy can be a powerful tool for overcoming suicidal tendencies while facing depression. Cognitive-behavioral therapy (CBT) and other forms of therapy can help individuals identify and change negative thought patterns, develop coping strategies, and improve overall mental health.

4. Build a support network: Having a strong support network can be crucial in overcoming suicidal tendencies while facing depression. This may include family members, friends, support groups, or mental health professionals.

5. Practice self-care: Taking care of oneself is important in managing depression and suicidal tendencies. This may include getting enough sleep, eating a healthy diet, getting regular exercise, and engaging in stress-reducing activities such as meditation or yoga.

6. Reduce access to lethal means: It is important to reduce access to lethal means such as firearms or medications. This may involve removing these items from the home, or ensuring that they are stored in a safe and secure location.

7. Create a safety plan: Creating a safety plan can help individuals manage suicidal thoughts and behaviors. A safety plan may include steps to take when experiencing suicidal thoughts, such as contacting a mental health professional or calling a crisis hotline.

Suicide is a devastating act that not only affects the individual but also has a profound impact on their loved ones, especially their parents. The pain and heartbreak that a parent experiences upon losing a child to suicide is indescribable. It is a wound that never fully heals, a burden that they carry with them for the rest of their lives.

Parents devote their entire lives to nurturing, caring for, and protecting their children. They invest their time, energy, and resources into raising their child to be a happy, healthy, and successful adult. They dream of seeing their child grow up, achieve their goals, and make a positive impact on the world.

When a child takes their own life, all of those dreams and aspirations are shattered. Parents are left with a profound sense of loss, guilt, and regret. They may blame themselves for not being able to prevent their child's suicide, even though it was not their fault. They may struggle with feelings of anger, confusion, and despair, wondering why their child felt so hopeless or alone that they saw no other way out.

The pain of losing a child to suicide is a burden that parents carry with them for the rest of their lives. It affects their mental and emotional well-being, their relationships, and their ability to find joy and meaning in life. It is a wound that never fully heals, a reminder of the pain and loss that they have endured.

So if you are struggling with thoughts of suicide, please remember that your parents love you deeply and want nothing more than to see you happy, healthy, and thriving. They would be devastated beyond measure if you were to take your own life. Reach out for help, talk to someone you trust, and remember that there is always hope. You are not alone, and there are people who care about you and want to support you through this difficult time.

Three

Re-framing Your Negative Thoughts: The Power of Positive Thinking

The human mind is a powerful tool that can shape our perception of reality. Thoughts and emotions play a crucial role in how we perceive the world around us, and negative thoughts can dampen our outlook and lead to feelings of stress, anxiety, and depression. Reframing negative thoughts and cultivating a positive mindset can have a profound impact on our mental and physical well-being. In this essay, we will explore the power of positive thinking and the benefits of reframing negative thoughts.

Negative thoughts are a natural part of human thinking. However, when we indulge in negative thoughts excessively, it begins to manifest in our lives. They can become a source of stress and anxiety, leading to an overall pessimistic outlook on life. Negative thoughts also tend to be self-perpetuating, which means the more we dwell on them, the more they consume us. This cycle of negative thinking can be broken by reframing our thoughts and creatively thinking positively.

Reframing is the process of consciously changing our perception of a situation. It is about taking a negative experience and consciously reinterpreting it in a more positive way. For example, suppose you receive negative feedback at work. In that case, a negative thought pattern may lead to self-doubt, anxiety, and a fear of being fired. Reframing this thought by taking it as constructive criticism and an opportunity for growth helps to re-frame and re-direct those negative thoughts.

Reframing can be challenging, especially when it comes to negative self-talk. We judge ourselves harshly and tend to magnify our weaknesses and downplay our strengths. Reframing negative self-talk is liberating as it frees us from the self-placed mental shackles, which weigh us down. To reframe negative thoughts about ourselves, we must identify why we take a critical view of ourselves and acknowledge that we are not alone in our self-judgment. Thus, instead of being stuck in negative feedback loops, we can encourage positive self-talk, which fosters self-esteem and a sense of well-being.

The power of positive thinking goes beyond just the psychological benefits. Positive thinking also plays a role in shaping physical health. Studies have shown that individuals with positive outlooks are more resilient to stress and are more likely to adopt a healthy lifestyle through consistent exercise and healthy eating. Additionally, positive thoughts can lead to lower blood pressure and a stronger immune system. Therefore, mental and physical well-being is intricately linked and is essential for an overall healthy lifestyle.

Our brain is an extremely complex organ that allows us to process information, make decisions and interact with our environment. It is made up of billions of neurons or nerve cells that communicate with each other through electrical and chemical signals. The connections between neurons are called synapses, and they are responsible for the transmission of information.

Rewiring the brain refers to the process of creating new neural pathways or changing existing ones. This can be achieved through a variety of ways, including training, therapy, meditation, and even medications. There are many benefits to rewiring the brain, including improved cognitive function, enhanced creativity, and better emotional regulation.

One of the most important factors in rewiring the brain is neuroplasticity. Neuroplasticity refers to the brain's ability to adapt and change throughout life, particularly in response to new experiences. This means that the brain is not a fixed entity but rather a malleable one that can be shaped and molded over time.

The process of rewiring the brain starts with the formation of new neural connections. This requires repeated practice and exposure to the desired activity or behavior. For example, if you want to learn a new skill like playing the piano, you need to practice regularly to create new neural pathways in your brain that support this skill.

Another way to rewiring the brain is through therapy, specifically cognitive-behavioral therapy (CBT). CBT focuses on changing negative thought patterns and behaviors by teaching individuals how to identify and challenge their negative thoughts. By changing these negative thought patterns, the brain can form new neural pathways that support positive behaviors and emotions.

Another technique for rewiring the brain is through meditation. Meditation has been shown to increase the thickness of the prefrontal cortex, the part of the brain responsible for attention and decision-making. It has also been shown to decrease activity in the amygdala, the part of the brain responsible for fear and anxiety.

Finally, medications can also help to rewiring the brain. For example, drugs used in the treatment of depression and anxiety work by changing the levels of neurotransmitters in the brain, which can help to create new neural pathways that support positive emotions and behaviors.

In conclusion, rewiring the brain is a complex process that requires dedication and persistence. However, the benefits of rewiring the brain are numerous, including improved cognitive function, enhanced creativity, and better emotional regulation. By understanding the principles of neuroplasticity and utilizing techniques such as therapy, meditation, and medication,etc.

Advantages of rewiring brain:

1. Enhanced Learning and Memory: The brain's ability to remember and learn is directly linked to its wiring. By rewiring your brain, you can improve its capacity to absorb and retain new information.

2. Improved Cognitive Function: Through exercises such as meditation and mindfulness, you can rewire your brain to improve focus, self-awareness, and overall cognitive function.

3. Improved Mental Health: Rewiring your brain can help reduce symptoms of depression, anxiety, and stress. By engaging in activities

that promote positive thinking and feelings, the brain can create new neural pathways that support healthier thought patterns.

4. Increased Resilience: Rewiring your brain can help increase resilience to stress and change. By practicing mindfulness and other techniques, you can change how your brain responds to stressful situations and build a more adaptable mindset.

5. Greater Creativity: Rewiring your brain can enhance creativity by enabling you to think more innovatively and see things from different perspectives. It can help generate new ideas and find unique solutions to problems.

There are many benefits of positive thinking including:

1. Increased resilience: Positive thinking can help you bounce back from setbacks and adapt to difficult situations with confidence.

2. Improved health: Studies have shown that positive thinking can reduce stress, lower blood pressure, boost the immune system, and even improve heart health.

3. Better relationships: Positive thinking can help you communicate effectively, build stronger connections with others, and resolve conflicts more easily.

4. Greater happiness: Focusing on the positive aspects of life can improve your overall mood and lead to greater feelings of joy and contentment.

5. Increased motivation: Positive thinking can help you set and achieve

goals, allowing you to stay motivated and focused on success.

6. Improved creativity: A positive mindset can lead to more innovative ideas and a greater willingness to take risks and try new things.

7. Enhanced mental alertness: Positive thinking can increase concentration, memory retention, and overall mental clarity.

Overall, positive thinking can lead to a more fulfilling and rewarding life, both personally and professionally

Overall, rewiring your brain can lead to many benefits .

Four

Understanding the mind body connection

The concept of the mind-body connection is based on the idea that our thoughts, emotions, and behaviors impact our physical health. For example, when we experience stress, we may have physical symptoms like headaches, stomachaches, and muscle tension. Similarly, when we feel sad or depressed, we may become physically fatigued or experience a lack of energy. Conversely, positive emotions like happiness and joy can have beneficial effects on our physical health by reducing stress levels and boosting our immune system.

The scientific community has conducted extensive research on the mind-body connection, and recent studies have shown that the connection is much more profound than previously thought. For instance, researchers have found that chronic stress can lead to physical conditions like heart disease, high blood pressure, and even cancer. When we experience stress, our bodies release hormones like cortisol, which can weaken our immune system and increase inflammation. Over time, chronic stress can cause lasting damage to our physical health.

On the other hand, studies have also shown that the mind-body connection can be used to improve our physical health. Techniques like meditation and mindfulness have been shown to reduce stress and improve overall well-being. In one study, patients with chronic pain who practiced mindfulness meditation reported a significant reduction in pain levels. Similarly, yoga has been found to reduce stress, improve flexibility, and lower blood pressure.

The mind-body connection also plays a crucial role in mental health. Mental illnesses like depression and anxiety can have profound effects on our physical health and vice versa. For instance, people with depression are more likely to experience physical symptoms like fatigue, headaches, and chronic pain. On the other hand, people with chronic pain or a physical illness are more likely to develop depression or anxiety. Addressing both the physical and emotional aspects of mental illness is essential for successful treatment and recovery.

In conclusion, the mind-body connection is a vital aspect of our overall health and well-being. Our thoughts, emotions, and behaviors impact our physical health, and vice versa. Chronic stress.

The mind and body connection is a powerful tool that can unlock numerous miraculous advantages. Here are some of the benefits that you can experience when your mind and body are in sync:

1. Improved Physical Health: When your mind is peaceful and your thoughts are positive, your body automatically responds positively. This reduces stress levels, boosts the immune system and reduces the risk of chronic illnesses.

2. Enhanced Mental Health: A strong mind-body connection can aid in mental wellness by reducing anxiety, depression, and preventing mood disorders.

3. Increased Energy: Practicing mind-body techniques such as yoga, meditation or tai chi, can help to increase your energy levels. These practices promote relaxation and deep breathing which can reduce fatigue throughout the day.

4. Better Sleep: Better sleep quality is possible with a mind-body connection. Deep breathing, relaxation techniques, and mindfulness can all improve sleep patterns.

5. Greater Resilience: Mind-body practices can build resilience which is important for navigating difficult situations in life.

6. Clarity of Thought: A healthy mind-body connection can clear out mental clutter, making space for improved focus and clarity of thought.

7. Boosted Creativity: Mind and body balance can unlock greater creativity and intuition.

8. Increased Confidence: Mind-body techniques boost self-esteem and confidence by decreasing negative self-talk, improving self-awareness, and promoting relaxation and positivity.

9. Better Relationships: The ability to be present in the moment and connect with others on a deeper level through empathy and compassion is increased with a healthy mind-body connection.

10. Spiritual Connection: A mind-body connection can help cultivate a

deeper sense of purpose, meaning and spirituality in life.

Proven psychological techniques to connect mind with body:

There are various psychological techniques that can help you connect your mind with your body. Some of them are:

1. Mindfulness meditation: This technique involves focusing on your breathing and paying attention to how your body feels in the present moment without judgment.

2. Progressive Muscle Relaxation (PMR): This technique involves tensing and relaxing specific muscle groups in your body while focusing on your breath, which enhances awareness of your physical sensations.

3. Body Scan Meditation: This technique involves focusing your attention on each part of your body, one at a time, to notice any physical sensations, feelings, or emotions that may be present.

4. Yoga: This practice involves combining physical postures, breathing exercises, and meditation to connect your mind and body.

5. Tai Chi: This slow and gentle Chinese martial art involves a series of flowing movements that improve balance, strengthen muscles, and reduce stress and anxiety.

6. Guided Imagery: This technique involves visualizing a calming, peaceful scene or scenario that helps you connect with your body and

reduce stress levels.

7. Biofeedback: This method uses electronic devices to monitor and provide feedback on your physiological responses and bodily functions, such as heart rate, blood pressure, and muscle tension to teach you how to control these functions with your mind.

Remember, it takes time and practice to develop mind-body awareness, so be patient and persistent in your efforts to connect your mind and body.

As good mental health can improve your life , may that be mental or physical . A negative mental approach can also ruin your life .

Mental problems can have significant effects on physical health. Here are some examples:

1. Chronic Stress: Prolonged stress caused by mental health issues, such as anxiety and depression, can lead to high blood pressure, heart disease, and digestive problems.

2. Insomnia: Mental health problems can cause insomnia, which in turn can increase the risk of obesity, diabetes, and cardiovascular disease.

3. Substance Abuse: Substance abuse and addiction can cause liver and kidney damage, brain damage, and other physical health problems.

4. Self-Harm: Self-harm behaviors, such as cutting or burning oneself, can lead to infections, scars, and other physical injuries.

5. Eating Disorders: Eating disorders, such as anorexia nervosa and bulimia, can cause malnutrition, osteoporosis, gastrointestinal problems, and other health complications.

6. Weakened Immune System: Mental health issues can weaken the immune system, making individuals more susceptible to infections and illnesses.

Overall, it is important to prioritize both mental and physical health to maintain a healthy overall well-being.

Importance of mental health:

Mental health is a crucial aspect of our overall well-being. It refers to our psychological, emotional, and social well-being, and it affects how we think, feel, and behave in our daily lives. It is essential to understand the importance of maintaining good mental health as it can have a significant impact on our quality of life.

One of the primary reasons why mental health is important is that it affects our physical health. Poor mental health has been linked to chronic health conditions like heart disease, diabetes, and obesity. This is because when we are stressed, anxious, or depressed, it can lead to unhealthy behaviors like overeating, smoking, and lack of physical activity. Hence, taking care of our mental health can help prevent such chronic conditions.

Moreover, good mental health also helps us lead fulfilling and satisfying lives. It enables us to cope with life's challenges, build resilience, and maintain healthy relationships. People with good mental health are more likely to be productive at work or school, have better social connections, and enjoy their leisure time.

Additionally, mental health issues can affect anyone, regardless of age, gender, or social status. According to the World Health Organization (WHO), one in four people in the world will be affected by a mental health disorder at some point in their lives. Therefore, understanding the importance of mental health and seeking help when needed can have a significant impact on our overall well-being.

In conclusion, mental health is an important aspect of our overall well-being, which cannot be neglected. Taking care of our mental health can enhance our physical health, improve our relationships, and enable us to lead fulfilling and satisfying lives. It is essential to prioritize our mental health and seek help when faced with mental health disorders.

Five

Learning to manage stress

Stress is a natural response of our body to any kind of change or threat in our environment. Though it can be beneficial at times, an excessive amount of stress can have adverse effects on our physical and mental health. It can cause anxiety, depression, high blood pressure, and heart diseases, among other things. Therefore, it is important to manage stress effectively to lead a happy and healthy life.

One of the first steps towards managing stress is to identify the source of stress. Once we know what is causing us stress, we can work towards resolving or reducing it. For instance, if work-related stress is affecting us, we can try to organize our workload, prioritize tasks, and take regular breaks to avoid burnout. If personal issues like financial problems are causing stress, we can try to seek help from financial advisors, create a budget plan, and implement it.

Another effective way to manage stress is through regular exercise. Exercise releases endorphins, which are natural mood boosters. It also distracts us from our problems and helps us feel more relaxed. Regular exercise can include simple activities like jogging, walking, cycling, swimming, or even yoga and meditation.

Having a good support system is also essential for managing stress. Friends, family, or professional counselors can provide emotional support and help us deal with the challenges we face. Socializing and interacting with others can help us relieve stress and make us feel more connected to those around us.

Engaging in hobbies or activities that we enjoy can also help us manage stress. It could be anything from reading books, cooking, gardening, painting, or playing musical instruments. Such activities help us switch off from our daily routine and provide a sense of fulfillment.

Moreover, taking care of our physical and emotional well-being is crucial in managing stress. Getting enough sleep, eating healthy, and avoiding unhealthy habits like smoking and excessive drinking can help reduce stress levels. Additionally, practicing relaxation techniques such as deep breathing exercises, listening to calming music, or trying aromatherapy can help us relax and reduce stress.

In conclusion, stress is an inevitable aspect of life, but it shouldn't control us. There are many ways to manage stress, and each person's approach may differ. By identifying the source of stress, exercising regularly, having a support system, engaging in hobbies, and taking care of our physical and emotional well-being, we can effectively manage stress and lead a happy and healthy life.

Major Causes of stress:

1. Work-related stress - heavy workloads, long working hours, conflicts with colleagues, lack of job security, difficult work relationships, etc.

2. Financial stress - financial instability, debts, inability to meet financial obligations, etc.

3. Relationship stress - problems with family, friends, and significant others, misunderstandings, disagreements, breakups, etc.

4. Health-related stress - chronic illnesses, injuries, disabilities, physical and mental health problems, etc.

5. Life transitions stress - major life changes such as moving, starting a new job, getting married, having a baby, divorce, etc.

6. Environmental stress - natural disasters, pollution, violent crimes, political unrest, social injustice, etc.

7. Personal stress - negative self-talk, perfectionism, self-doubt, low self-esteem, lack of purpose, etc.

8. Technological stress - overuse or dependency on technology, difficulty keeping up with technological advancements, fear of missing out, etc.

There are several techniques that can help you overcome stress quickly, including:

1. Deep breathing: Take deep breaths in through your nose for 5 seconds, hold it for another 5 seconds, and then slowly breathe out for another 5 seconds.

2. Progressive muscle relaxation: Tense up one muscle group at a time (e.g. fists, arms, shoulders, legs) for a few seconds, and then release them.

Repeat this for all muscle groups.

3. Visualization or guided imagery: Imagine yourself in a peaceful place, like a beach or a forest, and focus on the details of the surroundings.

4. Exercise: Take a quick walk or do a few stretching exercises to get your blood flowing and release endorphins.

5. Get organized: Make a to-do list or prioritize your tasks for the day. Knowing what you need to do can alleviate stress.

6. Talk to someone: Reach out to a friend or family member for support or talk to a therapist or counselor.

It's important to find what works best for you and to practice these techniques regularly to help overcome stress in the long run.

30 proven ways to manage stress:
1. Exercise regularly
2. Practice deep breathing techniques
3. Get enough rest and sleep
4. Maintain a healthy diet
5. Take breaks throughout the day
6. Stay organized and plan ahead
7. Learn time-management skills
8. Don't overcommit yourself
9. Prioritize your tasks
10. Talk to a professional if needed
11. Practice mindfulness meditation

12. Spend time in nature
13. Surround yourself with positive people
14. Laugh often
15. Listen to music
16. Take up a hobby or activity you enjoy
17. Reduce screen time
18. Avoid procrastination
19. Set realistic goals
20. Focus on what you can control
21. Practice relaxation techniques
22. Write in a journal
23. Take a hot bath or shower
24. Practice yoga or stretching
25. Volunteer or do something kind for others
26. Seek social support when needed
27. Avoid unhealthy coping mechanisms such as alcohol or drugs
28. Express your emotions in a healthy way
29. Find ways to make yourself laugh
30. Challenge negative thoughts and replace them with positive ones.

Overthinking can also help overcome stress
1. Overcoming overthinking can reduce anxiety and stress levels.
2. It can improve decision-making abilities.
3. It can increase productivity and efficiency.
4. It can improve relationships by reducing misunderstandings and miscommunications.
5. It can enhance creativity by allowing for more free-flowing thoughts.
6. It can improve overall mental health and well-being.

7. It can lead to a more positive outlook on life.
8. It can lead to increased self-confidence and self-esteem.
9. It can improve sleep quality.
10. It can lead to a more mindful and present lifestyle.

physiological proven techniques to calm mind:

Cognitive Restructuring: Changing Negative Thought Patterns

Progressive Muscle Relaxation: Relaxing Your Body to Calm Your Mind

Visualization Techniques: Using Imagery to Promote Relaxation

Breathing Exercises: Deep Breathing to Reduce Anxiety and Stress

Mindful Coloring: Using Art as a Tool for Relaxation and Mindfulness

Six

Overcoming trauma

O vercoming trauma refers to the process of healing and moving forward after experiencing a traumatic event or series of events. It involves acknowledging and processing the emotional and psychological impact of the trauma, as well as developing coping mechanisms to manage the symptoms of trauma. This can include seeking therapy, practicing self-care, and engaging in activities that promote healing and resilience. It is important to note that the process of overcoming trauma is unique to each individual and may take time, patience, and support from loved ones and mental health professionals.

Causes of trauma:

1. Neglect and emotional abuse: Trauma can result from experiences of neglect or emotional abuse, particularly in childhood. The experience

of being ignored, invalidated, or emotionally manipulated can cause long-lasting effects on an individual's mental health and wellbeing.

2. Immigration and refugee trauma: Trauma can result from experiences related to immigration or seeking asylum, such as being separated from family members, experiencing violence or persecution in one's home country, or facing discrimination and challenges in a new country.

3. Substance abuse and addiction: Trauma can result from experiences related to substance abuse or addiction, such as overdoses, witnessing or experiencing violence related to drug use, or experiencing addiction-related stigma and discrimination.

4. Medical trauma related to childbirth: Trauma can also result from experiences related to childbirth, such as traumatic births, complications during childbirth, or experiencing medical interventions without consent.

5. Trauma related to incarceration: Trauma can result from experiences related to incarceration, such as being incarcerated, witnessing or experiencing violence within the prison system, or experiencing discrimination and stigma related to a criminal record.

6.Acculturation trauma: Trauma can result from the process of adapting to a new culture, particularly for immigrants and refugees. This can include experiences of discrimination, feeling disconnected from one's cultural identity, and navigating cultural differences.

7. Interpersonal violence: Trauma can result from experiences of interpersonal violence, such as domestic violence, sexual assault, or stalking. These experiences can cause feelings of fear, shame, and

helplessness.

8.Trauma related to chronic illness: Trauma can result from experiences related to chronic illness, such as receiving a diagnosis, experiencing chronic pain, or facing limitations in daily life due to illness.

9.Trauma related to environmental disasters: Trauma can result from experiences related to environmental disasters, such as wildfires, hurricanes, or oil spills. These experiences can cause feelings of fear, loss, and uncertainty about the future.

10.Trauma related to law enforcement and criminal justice: Trauma can result from experiences related to law enforcement and criminal justice, such as experiencing police brutality, facing unjust sentencing or incarceration, or witnessing violence within the criminal justice system.

1. Acknowledging the trauma: The first step in overcoming trauma is acknowledging and accepting what has happened. This can be difficult, but it is an important part of the healing process.

2. Seeking support: It is important to seek support from a mental health professional, such as a therapist or counselor, who can help you work through the trauma and develop coping mechanisms.

3. Practicing self-care: Self-care is an essential part of overcoming trauma. This can include engaging in activities that promote relaxation and self-soothing, such as taking a warm bath or practicing mindfulness meditation.

4. Developing coping mechanisms: Coping mechanisms are strategies that help you manage the symptoms of trauma. This can include developing a routine, setting boundaries, and engaging in activities that promote a sense of safety and control.

5. Cultivating resilience: Resilience is the ability to bounce back from difficult experiences. Cultivating resilience involves building a support network, developing a positive outlook, and actively engaging in activities that promote personal growth and healing.

6. Addressing physical health: Trauma can have physical effects on the body, such as headaches, muscle tension, and fatigue. It is important to address these physical symptoms through exercise, healthy eating, and seeking medical care if necessary.

7. Processing emotions: Trauma can cause a range of emotions, including anger, guilt, and sadness. It is important to process these emotions in a healthy way, such as through journaling, talking to a loved one, or seeking therapy.

8. Building a support network: A strong support network can be essential in overcoming trauma. This can include friends, family, support groups, and mental health professionals.

9. Practicing self-compassion: It is important to be kind and compassionate to yourself during the healing process. This can involve practicing self-acceptance, self-forgiveness, and acknowledging your own strengths and resilience.

10. Finding meaning: While trauma can be a painful experience, it can also provide an opportunity for growth and personal transformation.

Finding meaning in the experience can help you move forward with a sense of purpose and hope.

11. Practicing grounding techniques: Grounding techniques can help you stay present and centered when you are experiencing symptoms of trauma, such as flashbacks or panic attacks. These techniques can include focusing on your breathing, using your senses to observe your surroundings, or repeating a mantra or affirmation.

12. Addressing negative beliefs: Trauma can cause negative beliefs about oneself or the world. It is important to address these negative beliefs and reframe them in a more positive and realistic way.

13. Setting goals: Setting goals can help you focus on the future and cultivate a sense of purpose after experiencing trauma. These goals can be small or large and can be related to any area of your life, such as career, relationships, or personal growth.

14. Using creative expression: Creative expression, such as art, music, or writing, can be a powerful tool for healing and self-expression. Engaging in creative activities can help you process emotions and express yourself in a safe and healthy way.

15. Practicing self-compassion: Self-compassion involves treating yourself with kindness, understanding, and acceptance. This can involve practicing self-care, setting boundaries, and acknowledging your own strengths and resilience.

Overcoming trauma is a complex and ongoing process that requires patience, self-care, and support. However, with the right tools and resources, it is possible to heal and move forward towards a brighter future. Remember, healing is a journey, not a destination, and it is important to be gentle and kind to yourself along the way.

Seven

Exploring your passion: hobbies and activities.

I t is important to note that finding the right hobby or activity for us may take some trial and error, and that it's okay to try different things until we find something that resonates with us. It's also important to make time for these activities in our daily or weekly routines, as they can provide a much-needed break from the stress and demands of everyday life.

Additionally, engaging in hobbies and activities can also help to promote a sense of purpose and meaning in our lives. When we have something to look forward to and work towards, it can help to improve our motivation and overall sense of fulfillment. This can lead to a more positive mindset, as we feel more confident and empowered in our ability to achieve our goals and pursue our passions.

Finally, it's important to remember that engaging in hobbies and activities should be a fun and enjoyable experience, rather than something that feels like a chore or obligation. By finding activities that we genuinely enjoy and look forward to, we can reap the many benefits that come with promoting a positive mindset and improving our mental health and well being.

Moreover, exploring hobbies and activities can also help us to develop new skills and interests that we may not have otherwise discovered. This can lead to personal growth and a sense of accomplishment, as we challenge ourselves to learn and try new things.

Furthermore, engaging in hobbies and activities can also help to reduce feelings of isolation and loneliness, which can have a negative impact on our mental health and well being. By connecting with others who share similar interests and passions, we can build new friendships and relationships that provide a sense of belonging and support.

In conclusion, exploring hobbies and activities can be a powerful tool for promoting a positive mindset and improving our mental health and well being. By finding activities that we enjoy and that provide us with a sense of purpose and fulfillment, we can reduce stress and anxiety, improve our mood, and build stronger connections with others. So, whether it's painting, running, volunteering, or practicing mindfulness, there are countless ways to explore our interests and passions and improve our mental health and well being in the process.

It's also important to remember that engaging in hobbies and activities doesn't have to be expensive or time-consuming. There are plenty of low-cost or free activities that we can explore, such as hiking, reading, or attending community events. Additionally, we can also find ways to incorporate our hobbies and interests into our daily routines, such as listening to music while we work or taking a walk during our lunch break.

Finally, if we're struggling to find hobbies or activities that resonate with us, it can be helpful to seek out support and guidance from a mental health professional or support group. They can provide us with resources and strategies for exploring our interests and passions, as well as help us to develop a positive mindset and improve our overall mental health and well being.

In summary, exploring hobbies and activities can be a powerful tool for promoting a positive mindset and improving our mental health and well being. By finding activities that we enjoy and that provide us with a sense of purpose and fulfillment, we can reduce stress and anxiety, improve our mood, build stronger connections with others, and develop new skills and interests. So, let's take some time to explore our passions and interests, and discover new ways to promote a positive mindset and improve our mental health and well being.

Another benefit of engaging in hobbies and activities is that it can help us to manage and cope with difficult emotions and experiences. For example, if we're struggling with anxiety or depression, engaging in activities that promote relaxation and mindfulness, such as yoga or meditation, can help to reduce symptoms and improve our overall mental health.

Moreover, hobbies and activities can also provide us with a sense of control and agency in our lives. When we engage in activities that we enjoy and that make us feel good, we're taking an active role in our own mental health and wellbeing. This can be especially empowering for those who may feel powerless or helpless in other areas of their lives.

Additionally, hobbies and activities can also help us to build resilience and cope with stress and adversity. By engaging in activities that challenge us and push us out of our comfort zones, we can develop a sense of confidence and strength that can help us to navigate difficult times in our lives.

In conclusion, engaging in hobbies and activities can have a multitude of benefits for our mental health and wellbeing. By finding activities that we enjoy and that provide us with a sense of purpose and fulfillment, we can reduce stress and anxiety, improve our mood, build stronger connections with others, develop new skills and interests, manage difficult emotions, and build resilience. So, let's make it a priority to explore our passions and interests, and discover new ways to promote a positive mindset and improve our mental health and well being.

Eight

Self love

Self-love is a concept that has become increasingly popular in recent years, and for good reason. It's the practice of treating ourselves with kindness, compassion, and respect, and it's essential for our mental health and well being. Self-love involves accepting ourselves as we are, flaws and all, and recognizing our own worth and value. It's about prioritizing our needs and desires, and taking care of ourselves in a way that promotes our happiness and fulfillment. In a world that often tells us we're not enough, practicing self-love is a radical act of defiance and a powerful tool for promoting a positive mindset and improving our overall well being.

When we practice self-love, we're essentially giving ourselves permission to be human and to make mistakes. We're acknowledging that we're not perfect, and that's okay. Instead of beating ourselves up for our flaws and shortcomings, we're learning to embrace them and to see them as a part of our unique and beautiful selves.

Moreover, self-love involves setting boundaries and saying no to things that don't serve us. It's about recognizing our own limits and needs, and taking steps to protect our mental and emotional health. This can include saying no to social events that drain our energy, or setting boundaries with people in our lives who may be toxic or harmful.

Additionally, self-love is about practicing self-care in a way that feels authentic and meaningful to us. This can include anything from taking a relaxing bath, to going for a walk in nature, to indulging in a favorite hobby or activity. By taking care of ourselves in this way, we're sending a message to ourselves that we're worthy of love and attention, and that our needs matter.

In conclusion, self-love is a powerful practice that can have a trans formative effect on our mental health and well being. By treating ourselves with kindness, compassion, and respect, we're promoting a positive mindset and building a strong foundation for our overall health and happiness. So, let's make self-love a priority in our lives, and learn to embrace and celebrate all that makes us unique and wonderful.

Starting to practice self-love can be a challenging process, especially if we're used to being self-critical or neglecting our own needs. However, there are some simple steps that we can take to begin cultivating a more loving and compassionate relationship with ourselves.

Firstly, it's important to start with self-awareness. We can begin by paying attention to the thoughts and feelings that arise within us, and noticing when we're being overly critical or judgmental of ourselves. By becoming aware of these patterns, we can start to challenge them and replace them with more positive and affirming thoughts.

Secondly, we can make a conscious effort to prioritize our own needs and desires. This can include setting aside time for self-care activities, such as exercise, meditation, or spending time in nature. It can also involve learning to say no to things that don't serve us, and setting boundaries with others in our lives.

Thirdly, we can practice self-compassion by treating ourselves with the kindness and understanding that we would offer to a close friend or loved one. This involves acknowledging our own struggles and challenges, and recognizing that we're doing the best we can in any given moment.

Finally, it can be helpful to seek out support from others, such as a therapist, support group, or trusted friend or family member. By connecting with others who share our struggles and challenges, we can feel less alone and more supported in our journey towards self-love.

In conclusion, starting to practice self-love can be a transformative process that can have a profound impact on our mental health and well being. By becoming more self-aware, prioritizing our own needs, practicing self-compassion, and seeking out support from others, we can begin to cultivate a more loving and compassionate relationship with ourselves.

There are many different methods and practices that can help us to cultivate self-love and compassion. Here are a few examples:

1. Positive self-talk: One of the most effective ways to practice self-love is to speak to ourselves in a positive and affirming way. This can involve identifying and challenging negative self-talk, and replacing it with more positive and empowering statements. For example, instead

of saying "I'm not good enough," we can say "I am worthy and deserving of love and respect."

2. Self-care: Practicing self-care is an essential component of self-love. This can involve taking care of our physical, emotional, and spiritual needs, such as getting enough sleep, eating nourishing foods, exercising regularly, and engaging in activities that bring us joy and fulfillment.

3. Mindfulness: Mindfulness is the practice of being present and fully engaged in the current moment. By cultivating mindfulness, we can learn to observe our thoughts and feelings without judgment, and develop a greater sense of self-awareness and self-compassion. Practices such as meditation, yoga, and deep breathing can be helpful in cultivating mindfulness.

4. Gratitude: Practicing gratitude is another powerful tool for cultivating self-love and compassion. By focusing on the things in our lives that we're grateful for, we can shift our attention away from negative thoughts and feelings, and develop a greater sense of appreciation for ourselves and our lives.

5. Seeking support: Finally, seeking support from others is an important part of practicing self-love. This can involve connecting with a therapist, joining a support group, or reaching out to trusted friends or family members. By sharing our struggles and challenges with others, we can feel less alone and more supported in our journey towards self-love.

Self-love is essential for our overall mental health and well being. Here are some important reasons why self-love is so crucial:

1. Boosts self-esteem: When we practice self-love, we're essentially

acknowledging our own worth and value. This can help to boost our self-esteem and confidence, and promote a more positive self-image.

2. Reduces stress and anxiety: Practicing self-love can help to reduce stress and anxiety by promoting a more positive and compassionate mindset. When we treat ourselves with kindness and compassion, we're less likely to get caught up in negative thoughts and feelings.

3. Improves relationships: When we love and accept ourselves, we're better able to love and accept others. By cultivating self-love, we can improve our relationships with others by becoming more compassionate, empathetic, and understanding.

4. Increases resilience: Self-love can help to increase our resilience in the face of challenges and setbacks. When we have a strong sense of self-love and self-worth, we're better able to bounce back from difficult situations and to persevere through adversity.

5. Promotes self-care: Practicing self-love involves taking care of ourselves in a way that promotes our overall health and well being. By prioritizing self-care, we can improve our physical, emotional, and spiritual health, and feel more energized and fulfilled in our daily lives.

Nine

Part of music in life

Music is an integral part of human culture and has been present in all societies throughout history. It is a universal language that transcends cultural and linguistic barriers, and has the power to connect people, evoke emotions, and enhance our daily lives in countless ways. From the earliest forms of music created by our ancestors to the modern music industry, music has played a vital role in human life, and has been used for a variety of purposes, including religious, social, cultural, and therapeutic. In this essay, we will explore the importance of music in our daily lives, and examine the many unique and valuable ways in which it can impact our mental, emotional, and physical well-being.

Music has the ability to evoke strong emotions and memories, and can be used as a tool for self-expression and communication. Whether we're listening to music, singing, playing an instrument, or dancing, music can help us to connect with ourselves and others on a deeper level. Moreover, music has been shown to have many positive effects on our mental and physical health. For example, listening to music can help to reduce stress and anxiety, improve mood, boost cognitive function, and promote relaxation and sleep.

In addition, music has played a vital role in shaping our cultural identity and history. From traditional folk music to contemporary pop and hip-hop, music reflects the diverse and complex nature of human experience, and has been used to express ideas, beliefs, and values throughout history. Music has also been a powerful tool for social and political change, and has been used to raise awareness about important issues and to bring people together to effect change

Music is a universal language that has the power to connect people, evoke emotions, and enhance our daily lives in countless ways. Here are some unique and important ways in which music can impact our lives:

1. Promotes creativity: Music has the power to inspire creativity and imagination in people of all ages. Whether we're listening to music or creating our own, music can help to unlock our creative potential and encourage us to think outside the box.

2. Enhances mood: Music has been shown to have a powerful impact on our mood and emotions. Whether we're feeling happy, sad, or somewhere in between, music can help us to process our emotions and feel more connected to ourselves and others.

3. Improves cognitive function: Music has been linked to improved cognitive function, including memory, attention, and language skills. Listening to music can help to stimulate the brain and promote learning and brain development.

4. Reduces stress and anxiety: Music has a calming effect on the body and can help to reduce stress and anxiety. Listening to music or playing an instrument can help to lower heart rate and blood pressure, and promote relaxation and overall well-being.

5. Fosters community: Music has the power to bring people together and foster a sense of community and connection. Whether we're attending a concert, playing in a band, or simply listening to music with friends, music can help to create meaningful and lasting connections with others.

Here are some ways in which music can help to heal us emotionally:

1. Elicits emotional responses: Music has the ability to elicit strong emotional responses in listeners. Whether we're listening to a sad ballad or an upbeat dance track, music can help us to connect with our emotions and process them in a healthy way.

2. Acts as a form of self-expression: Music can be used as a form of self-expression and can help us to communicate our thoughts and feelings in a way that is creative and meaningful. Whether we're writing our own music or simply listening to music that resonates with us, music can help us to express ourselves and feel heard and understood.

3. Promotes relaxation and stress reduction: Listening to calming music can help to reduce stress and promote relaxation. Music has been shown to lower heart rate and blood pressure, and can help us to feel more calm and centered in the midst of challenging situations.

4. Boosts mood and promotes positive emotions: Music has the ability to boost mood and promote positive emotions. Listening to upbeat

music can help us to feel more energized and motivated, while listening to soothing music can help us to feel more calm and content.

5. Enhances social connections: Music can help to enhance social connections and promote a sense of community. Whether we're attending a concert or simply listening to music with friends, music can bring people together and foster a sense of belonging and connection.

6.Music can reduce stress and anxiety: Listening to relaxing music can help to lower our heart rate and blood pressure, and reduce the levels of stress hormones in our body. This can promote a sense of calm and relaxation, and help us to feel more grounded and centered.

7.Music can improve mood: Listening to upbeat music can help to boost our mood and energy levels, and promote feelings of happiness and positivity. This can be especially helpful when we're feeling down or depressed, and can help to lift our spirits and improve our outlook on life.

8.Music can help us to process emotions: Music can help us to connect with our emotions and express them in a safe and healthy way. Whether we're listening to sad music to help us grieve, or upbeat music to help us celebrate, music can provide a powerful outlet for our emotions.

9.Music can promote self-reflection: Music can help us to reflect on our thoughts and feelings, and gain a deeper understanding of ourselves. Whether we're listening to music that speaks to our personal experiences, or creating our own music to express our innermost thoughts and feelings, music can help us to connect with ourselves on a deeper level.

10. Music can promote social connection: Music can bring people together and promote a sense of community and connection. Whether we're attending a concert, singing in a choir, or playing in a band, music can help us to connect with others who share our interests and passions.

In conclusion, music has the power to heal us emotionally in countless ways. Whether we're listening to music for pleasure, using music as a tool for self-expression and reflection, or connecting with others through music, music can help us to process our emotions, reduce stress and anxiety, improve our mood, and promote a sense of wellbeing and connection. So, let's continue to explore the many unique and valuable ways in which music can impact our emotional health, and celebrate the power and beauty of this universal language.

Ten

Gratitude and positivity

Gratitude and positivity are two essential components of a happy and fulfilling life. Gratitude is the act of acknowledging and appreciating the good things in our lives, while positivity is the mindset of focusing on the positive aspects of our experiences and looking for the good in every situation. These two concepts are closely intertwined, and can have a profound impact on our mental, emotional, and physical well-being. In this essay, we will explore the importance of gratitude and positivity, and examine the many unique and valuable ways in which they can improve our lives and help us to achieve greater happiness and fulfillment.

At its core, gratitude is about recognizing the good things in our lives and expressing appreciation for them. This can include anything from the people we love, to the opportunities we have, to the simple pleasures of everyday life. When we practice gratitude regularly, we cultivate a sense of abundance and contentment, and become more aware of the many blessings in our lives. This, in turn, can help us to feel happier, more fulfilled, and more connected to the world around us.

Positivity, on the other hand, is about looking for the good in every situation, and focusing on the positive aspects of our experiences. This doesn't mean ignoring the challenges or difficulties we face, but rather, approaching them with a mindset of optimism and resilience. When we cultivate a positive mindset, we become more resilient in the face of adversity, and are better able to handle stress and uncertainty. We also become more open to new experiences and opportunities, and are more likely to find joy and meaning in our lives.

Negative thoughts are a common experience for many people, and can have a significant impact on our mental and emotional wellbeing. There are many different factors that can contribute to negative thoughts, including:

1. Past experiences: Negative experiences from our past can leave a lasting impact on our thoughts and emotions. Traumatic events, such as abuse or neglect, can create negative thought patterns that persist long after the event has ended.

2. Environmental factors: Our environment can also play a role in shaping our thoughts and emotions. Living in a stressful or chaotic environment, for example, can lead to negative thoughts and feelings.

3. Genetics: Some people may be genetically predisposed to negative thoughts and emotions. Research has shown that certain genes may be linked to depression and anxiety.

4. Chemical imbalances: Chemical imbalances in the brain can

also contribute to negative thoughts and emotions. Imbalances in neurotransmitters such as serotonin, dopamine, and norepinephrine can lead to feelings of sadness, anxiety, and hopelessness.

5. Negative self-talk: The way we talk to ourselves can also impact our thoughts and emotions. Negative self-talk, such as telling ourselves we're not good enough or that we'll never succeed, can create a cycle of negative thinking.

6. Stress: Chronic stress can also contribute to negative thoughts and emotions. When we're under constant stress, our brains release cortisol, a hormone that can lead to feelings of anxiety and depression.

It's important to recognize that negative thoughts are a normal part of the human experience, and that everyone experiences them from time to time. However, if negative thoughts are impacting your quality of life, it may be helpful to seek support from a mental health professional.

Eleven

Loving life : realizing the beauty of life

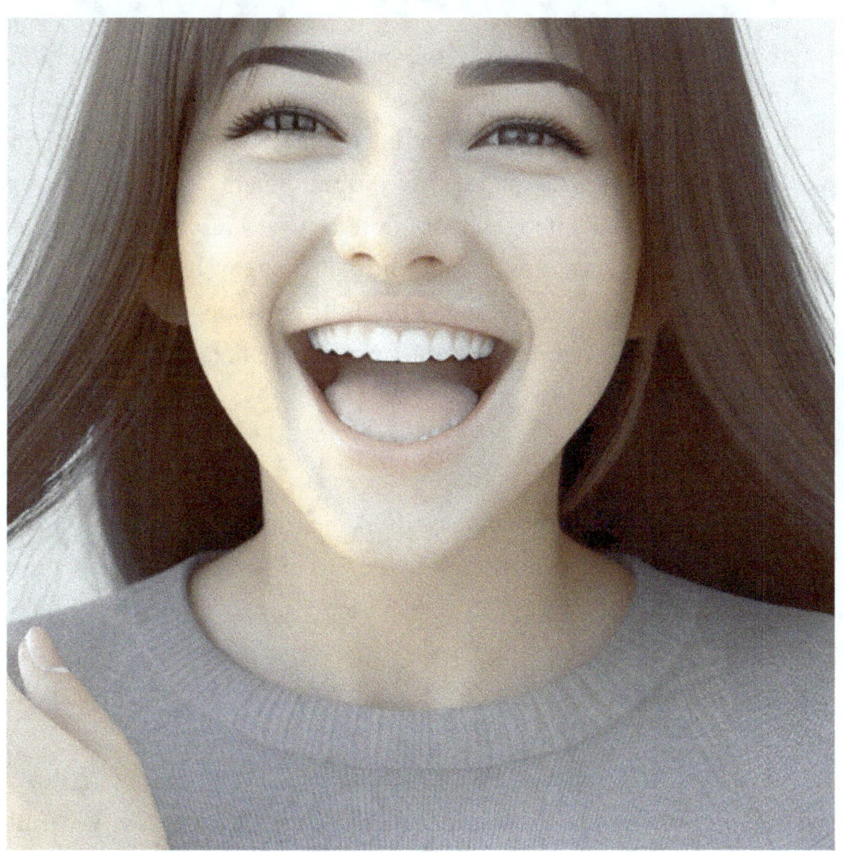

Loving life is a concept that encompasses a deep appreciation and gratitude for the gift of life. It is about finding joy and meaning in everyday experiences, and embracing the challenges and opportunities that come our way. Loving life is not just about feeling happy all the time, but about cultivating a sense of purpose, connection, and fulfillment in our lives. It involves recognizing the beauty and wonder of the world around us, and taking the time to savor the simple pleasures of life. In this fast-paced and often stressful world, loving life can be a powerful antidote to stress, anxiety, and depression. By embracing a mindset of love and gratitude, we can transform our lives and find greater happiness and fulfillment.

Loving life means appreciating the beauty of existence and making the most of every moment. It involves cultivating a positive outlook, embracing new experiences, and finding joy in the simple things. When we love life, we feel a sense of purpose and fulfillment, and we are better able to handle the challenges that come our way. Loving life is not always easy, but it is a worthwhile pursuit that can bring us greater happiness, contentment, and meaning. In this article, we will explore some of the ways in which we can learn to love life and find greater fulfillment in our daily lives.

Life is undoubtedly short and beautiful. The time we are given on this earth is precious and fleeting, and it is up to us to make the most of it. Every moment is an opportunity to experience joy, love, and connection with others. Life is a gift, and we should cherish it and make the most of the time we have.

There is so much to appreciate and enjoy in life. The beauty of nature, the laughter of friends, the warmth of a loving embrace - these are all experiences that make life worth living. Even in the face of challenges and adversity, there is always something to be grateful for.

Unfortunately, it is all too easy to get caught up in the stresses and distractions of daily life. We can become so focused on our goals and ambitions that we forget to appreciate the beauty of the present moment. We can become so consumed by our anxieties and fears that we forget to savor the simple pleasures of life.

It is important to remember that life is short, and we should make the most of it. We should prioritize the things that truly matter - our relationships, our passions, and our sense of purpose. We should take risks, try new things, and pursue our dreams with passion and determination.

When we realize the true value of life, we start to appreciate the little things that we often take for granted. A simple hug from a loved one, a beautiful sunset, a smile from a stranger - these small moments can bring so much joy and meaning to our lives.

It's important to remember that life is not just about achieving success or accumulating material possessions. While these things can be important, they are not the ultimate source of happiness and fulfillment. True happiness comes from within, from cultivating a sense of purpose, passion, and connection with others.

In the end, we will all leave this world behind. But what matters is how we lived our lives while we were here. Did we make a positive impact on those around us? Did we pursue our passions and dreams with courage and determination? Did we love deeply and live fully?

Life is short and beautiful, and we should make the most of it. We should embrace every moment with gratitude and joy, and seek to live a life that inspires others and leaves a lasting legacy of love and kindness.

We should fully love our life without worrying about society because it is our own unique journey, and we deserve to live it on our own terms. Society often imposes rigid expectations and standards that can limit our freedom and creativity, and prevent us from fully expressing ourselves. We may feel pressured to conform to certain norms or expectations, even if they are not in alignment with our true selves.

But when we let go of these societal expectations and embrace our own individuality, we open ourselves up to a world of possibility and joy. We can pursue our passions, follow our dreams, and live a life that is true to our deepest values and desires. We can connect with others who share our vision and values, and create a community of like-minded individuals who support and uplift each other.

It can be scary to step outside of the box and pursue our own path, but it is worth it. When we fully embrace our life and ourselves, we experience a deep sense of joy and fulfillment that cannot be found in conformity or approval-seeking. We become more resilient, more creative, and more authentic in our relationships and endeavors.

It is important to remember that we only have one life to live, and we should make the most of it. We should not let society's expectations or judgments hold us back from living a life that is true to ourselves. We should fully love our life and embrace every moment with gratitude and joy, knowing that we are living our own unique journey in the way that feels most authentic and fulfilling to us.

When we fully love our life, we also become more compassionate and understanding towards others. We begin to see the beauty and uniqueness in every individual, and we appreciate the diversity and richness of the world around us. We become more open-minded and accepting of different ways of life and perspectives, and we learn to connect with others on a deeper level.

Furthermore, fully loving our life allows us to make a positive impact on the world around us. When we follow our passions and pursue our dreams, we can inspire others to do the same. We can use our unique talents and strengths to make a difference in the lives of others, whether it be through art, music, activism, or any other avenue that speaks to our soul.

Ultimately, fully loving our life is a radical act of self-love and self-care. It is a way of honoring ourselves and our journey, and embracing the fullness of our humanity. It is a way of breaking free from the limitations and constraints of society, and living a life that is authentic, fulfilling, and joyful.

So let us fully love our life, without worrying about society's expectations or judgments. Let us embrace our unique journey with open hearts and minds, and live a life that is true to ourselves. Let us inspire others to do the same, and create a world that is more compassionate, creative, and joyful for all.

Our parents are the first and most enduring source of love in our lives. From the moment we are born, they shower us with affection and care, nurturing us and helping us grow into the person we are meant to be. Their love is unconditional and unwavering, a constant presence in our lives that gives us strength, comfort, and support.

As we grow older, we may take their love for granted, assuming that it will always be there. But the truth is that our parents' love is one of the most precious gifts we will ever receive. It is a love that is selfless, sacrificial, and enduring, a love that is willing to make any sacrifice for our happiness and well-being.

Our parents' love is precious because it is a reflection of the best of humanity. It is a love that is rooted in the deepest values of compassion, kindness, and generosity. It is a love that inspires us to be our best selves, to live with integrity and purpose, and to make a positive impact on the world.

When we fully appreciate the preciousness of our parents' love, we are filled with a sense of gratitude and awe. We realize that we are blessed beyond measure to have such wonderful, loving parents in our lives, and we cherish every moment we have with them.

So let us honor and cherish the precious love of our parents. Let us express our gratitude and love to them every chance we get, and let us strive to live our lives in a way that honors the sacrifices and selflessness of their love. For in doing so, we honor the best of humanity and create a legacy of love that will endure for generations to come.

* * *

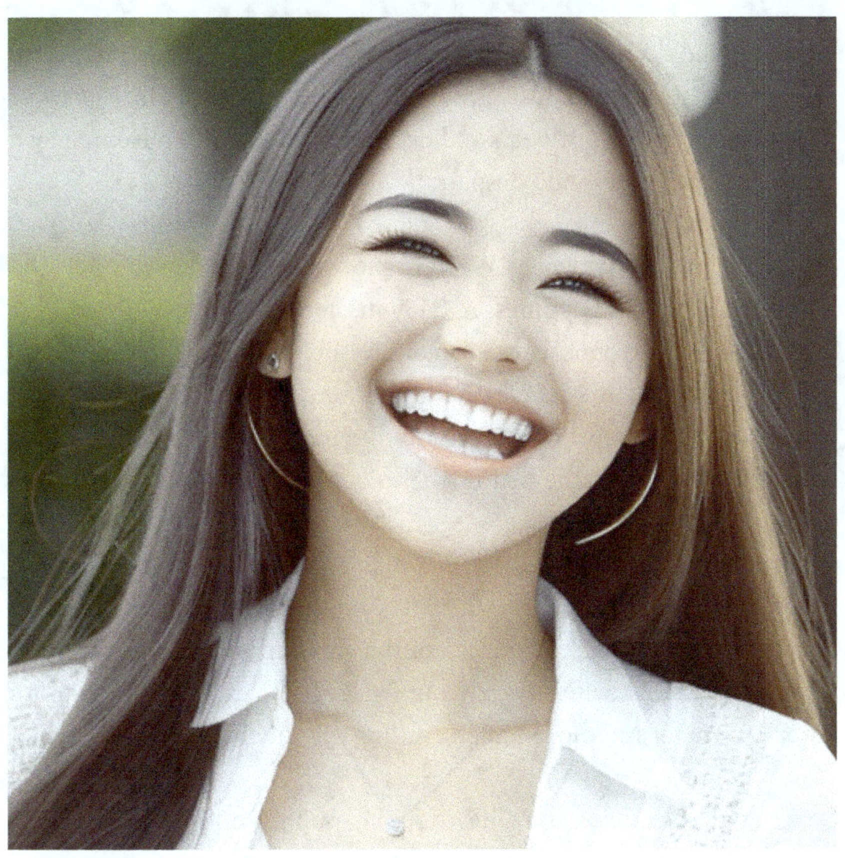

Life is a precious gift, filled with endless possibilities, experiences, and opportunities. It is a journey that is unique to each of us, filled with its own challenges, triumphs, and moments of beauty. Yet, so many of us waste this precious gift by succumbing to depression and despair, robbing ourselves of the joy, love, and happiness that life has to offer.

The truth is that life is meant to be lived fully, with passion, purpose, and love. We are meant to connect with others, to find meaning and purpose in our work, to explore the world around us, and to experience the full range of emotions that make us human.

When we allow depression to take hold of our lives, we cut ourselves off from these experiences and opportunities. We isolate ourselves from others, lose sight of our goals and dreams, and become consumed by a sense of hopelessness and despair.

But there is another way. We can choose to love our life and the people in it, to find happiness and joy in the midst of even the darkest moments. We can choose to reach out for help, to connect with others who understand our struggles and can offer support and guidance. We can choose to pursue our passions, to find meaning and purpose in our work, and to create a life that is true to our deepest values and desires.

When we choose to love our life and the people in it, we open ourselves up to a world of possibility and joy. We begin to see the beauty in the world around us, to appreciate the small moments of grace and kindness that make life worth living. We become more resilient, more compassionate, and more understanding of ourselves and others.

So let us choose to love our life, to find happiness and joy in the midst of even the darkest moments. Let us reach out for help when we need it, and connect with others who can offer support and guidance. Let us pursue our passions, find meaning and purpose in our work, and create a life that is true to our deepest values and desires. For in doing so, we honor the precious gift of life and create a legacy of love and happiness that will endure for generations to come.

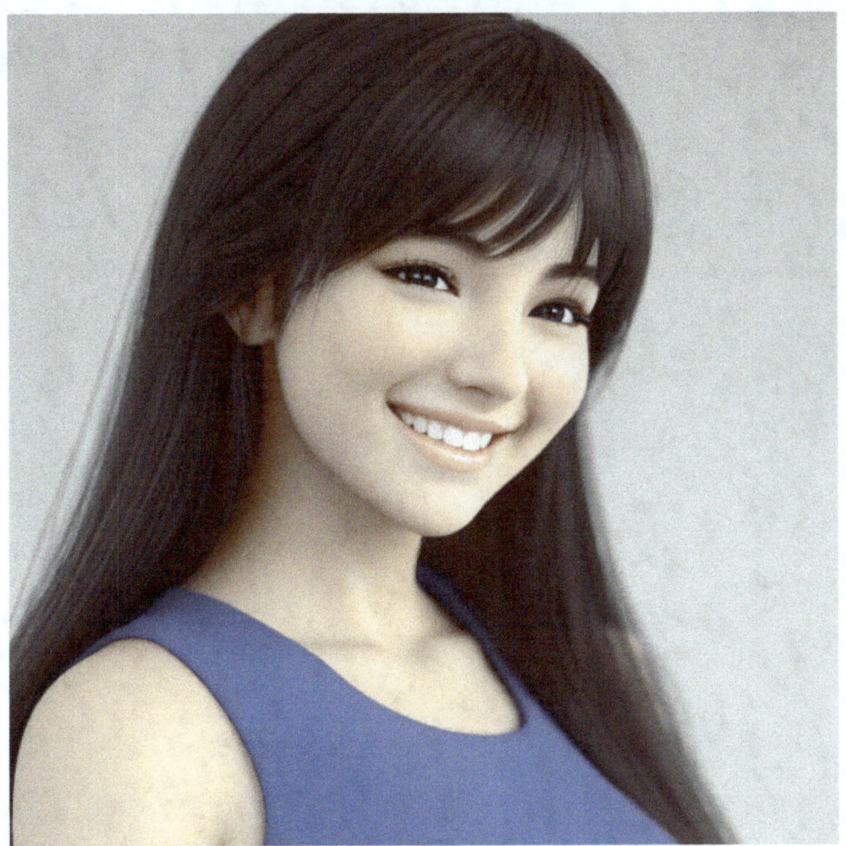

Life is beautiful , it's too short to waste it in being depressed so leave your life to the fullest because, you never know if would wake up tomorrow to see this beautiful life or not ...!

(✳✳)